MARGARET NEWMAN

Notes on Nursing Theories

SERIES EDITORS

Chris Metzger McQuiston
Doctoral Candidate, Wayne State University

Adele A. Webb
College of Nursing, University of Akron

Notes on Nursing Theories is a series of monographs designed to provide the reader with a concise description of conceptual frameworks and theories in nursing. Each monograph includes a biographical sketch of the theorist, origin of the theory, assumptions, concepts, propositions, examples for application to practice and research, a glossary of terms, and a bibliography of classic works, critiques, and research.

1   **Martha Rogers: The Science of Unitary Human Beings**
    Louette R. Johnson Lutjens

2   **Imogene King: A Conceptual Framework for Nursing**
    Christina L. Sieloff Evans

3   **Callista Roy: An Adaptation Model**
    Louette R. Johnson Lutjens

4   **Dorothea Orem: Self-Care Deficit Theory**
    Donna L. Hartweg

5   **Rosemarie Parse: Theory of Human Becoming**
    Sheila Bunting

6   **Margaret Newman: Health as Expanding Consciousness**
    Joanne Marchione

7   **Paterson and Zderad: Humanistic Nursing Theory**
    Nancy O'Connor

8   **Madeleine Leininger: Cultural Care Diversity and Universality Theory**
    Cheryl L. Reynolds and Madeleine M. Leininger

9   **Florence Nightingale: An Environmental Adaptation Theory**
    Louise C. Selanders

10 **Hildegard E. Peplau: Interpersonal Nursing Theory**
    Cheryl Forchuk

11 **Betty Neuman: The Neuman Systems Model**
    Karen S. Reed

12 **Ida Jean Orlando: A Nursing Process Theory**
    Norma Jean Schmieding

MARGARET NEWMAN

Health as Expanding Consciousness

Joanne Marchione

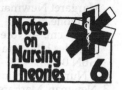

Notes
on
Nursing
Theories
6

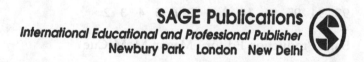

SAGE Publications
International Educational and Professional Publisher
Newbury Park   London   New Delhi

For information address:

SAGE Publications, Inc.
2455 Teller Road
Newbury Park, California 91320

SAGE Publications Ltd.
6 Bonhill Street
London EC2A 4PU
United Kingdom

SAGE Publications India Pvt. Ltd.
M-32 Market
Greater Kailash I
New Delhi 110 048 India

Printed in the United States of America

Library of Congress Cataloging-in-Publication Data

Marchione, Joanne M.
    Margaret Newman: Health as expanding consciousness / Joanne
Marchione.
        p.   cm.—(Notes on nursing theories; v. 6)
    Includes bibliographical references.
    ISBN 0-8039-4796-8.—ISBN 0-8039-4797-6 (pbk.)
    1. Nursing—Philosophy. 2. Health—Philosophy.
3. Newman, Margaret A. 4. Consciousness. I. Newman, Margaret A.
Health as expanding consciousness. II. Title. III. Series.
RT84.5.M36 1993   92-32000
613—dc20   CIP

93 94 95 96 10 9 8 7 6 5 4 3 2

Sage Production Editor: Megan M. McCue

Contents

Foreword, *Jean Watson*   vii

Preface   x

Acknowledgments   xii

Biographical Sketch of the Nurse Theorist   1

1. Origin of the Theory   3

2. Assumptions of the Theory   5
   Explicit Assumptions   5
   Implicit Assumptions   6

3. Concepts of the Theory   7
   Consciousness   8
   Time-Space   8
   Movement   9
   Pattern Recognition   10
   Pattern   11
   Expanding Consciousness   11

4. Newman's Theory and Nursing's Paradigm
   Concepts   12
   Person   13
   Environment   13
   Health   13
   Nursing   14

5. Propositions   15

6. Overview of Newman's Theory   17

7. Evolving the Pattern of the Whole   21
    A Case Study: Client K   21

8. Framework for Assessing the Pattern of the Whole   25
    A Case Study: Client X   26

9. Newman's Theory and Family Health   33

10. Research and Newman's Theory   34

11. Conclusion   38

    Glossary   39

    References   44

    Bibliography   47

    About the Author   51

Foreword

I believe Margaret Newman's theory of health is the latest turn in nursing theory and represents some of the most astute thinking in contemporary nursing. In 1987, I was honored to review her book *Health as Expanding Consciousness* (Watson, 1987), which laid out her evolving theory. Now I am equally honored to do the foreword to Joanne Marchione's fine monograph of Newman's work.

As Newman continues to take nursing significant steps forward in transforming the old paradigm of science, nursing, and health into the new world of science, nursing, and health, Marchione's clear application of the theory to individual, family, and community health praxis helps us reach yet another level of evolution and "expanding consciousness" with respect to Newman's work.

Marchione's work reflects several years of continuous experimentation and application of Newman's theory whereby she has had the opportunity to change as the theory has changed. Thus, this book comes after Marchione's sustained theoretical and experiential inquiry and dialogue with the nurse theorist. As such, it represents the latest thinking and translation of Newman's concepts of consciousness, time-space, movement, pattern recognition, pattern, and health as expanding consciousness, to praxis.

Marchione's lucid and succinct overview of Newman's theory provides both a summary and an intepretation of the theory as well as a conceptual translation that allows one to apply all of the theoretical assumptions and key concepts. She makes the theory live and breath through her straightforward presentation of case studies that transfer theoretical concepts of "pattern of the whole" to concrete application to individual and family health.

The discussion on praxis research provides an informed, contemporary perspective on the nature of appropriate, productive, and congruent research and methods of inquiry related to Newman's (and others) evolving theory. Marchione's experience and examples invite dialogue with the reader; this, in turn, has the effect of modeling both theory and method through the author-reader exchange that compiles the narrative for the text. This very process thereby mirrors the theory and praxis method being presented. Thus, in an indirect way, engaging with the ideas in the book becomes an exemplar of the very theory of expanding consciousness, which in turn has the effect of verifying and experientially validating the theory.

This work offers a special invitation for nurses and nursing to come into a new unitary relationship with theory, research, and clinical practice—a form of praxis and process that is dialogic, narrative, and evolving. To come into a new expanding health consciousness—consciousness that is evolving and whole. To come into a new form of holographic science that is pattern laden and unfolding. To come into a new form of nursing that is informed by consciousness, by process, by health and wholeness—a new form of nursing that is overtly value laden and continuous in time and space, yet transcendent of time and space. To come into a new convergence of nursing theory and nursing assessment and praxis that is choosing, communicating, exchanging, feeling, knowing, moving, perceiving, relating, and valuing of process, pattern, and expanding health consciousness. All of these "coming togethers" in Marchione's book help one to see the importance of Margaret Newman's contribution to nursing and the spin-offs her work is bringing to the nursing profession and to the broader health sciences.

The intellectual and praxis excitement of Newman's and Marchione's work is that they are open, in process, and ready to discover new patterns; they are receptive to exchange to allow emergence of the whole to unfold as this theory continues to evolve. We are all invited to participate in this excitement of unfolding, evolution, and discovery in our unitary transformative praxis of health as expanding consciousness.

JEAN WATSON, RN, PHD, FAAN
Professor of Nursing and
Director of The Center for Human Caring,
University of Colorado, Health Sciences Center,
Denver, Colorado

Preface

Theory development in nursing is the process by which the discipline of nursing is respected as a science and is recognized for its special focus on health and human caring.

In recent times, several nurse theorists have developed diverse and respected models and theories for nursing, thus contributing to the advancement of nursing science.

Margaret Newman is one of several internationally renowned nursing theorists who have led the way in the development of nursing science. A current description of Dr. Newman's theory of health is set forth in this text. The concepts, propositions, assumptions, and practice/research applications of the theory are summarized and presented, with the advice that this book is to be viewed as a supplement to Newman's (1979, 1986) primary texts. Primary and recent writings that explicate her theory can be found in the bibliography provided in this book. The references and sources cited in the bibliography serve as means to encourage additional reading.

This text of Newman's theory of health is one of several in a series, *Notes on Nursing Theories*, from Sage Publications. The intent of this text is to assist students in nursing to clarify concepts, identify assumptions, relate propositions, and understand practice/research applications of Newman's theory. Nursing faculty may also find this text useful for a succinct and current review of Newman's theory of health.

My sincere thanks are extended to Dr. Margaret Newman, who so generously consented to review and critique a draft of this text prior to its publication. I am especially grateful to Dr. Newman for encouraging me to engage in an independent study with her at The Pennsylvania State University in 1983, and for her continued support and encouragement over the past several years.

A special thank-you is extended to Associate Professor Susan Stearns, M.S.N., of the College of Nursing, University of Akron. Her gentle advice and sensitive critiques of several drafts of this text have been vital to the completion of this project.

JOANNE MARCHIONE

Acknowledgments

For my family and friends.

In honor of the memories of my father, my Uncle Tony, and Alfalfa. The spirit and essence of each of these three special relatives were with me as I moved, in an ever-expanding consciousness, to complete this project.

In gratitude for their unconditional love, loyal friendship, and energizing encouragement, I dedicate this book to my mother, to Tony III, Anthony, Dean, Gloria, Ruby, Pauline, Adam, Angie, Camille, Gregory, Cindy, Sally, Dianne, Lori, Pam, Terri, Bradley, Mark, Ben, Echo, Sandie, Dustin, Erin, Susan, June, Mary, Bob, Gharith, and there are many others.

Biographical Sketch of the Nurse Theorist:
Margaret Newman, RN, PhD, FAAN

Born: 1933

Current Position: Professor, School of Nursing, University of Minnesota; Nurse theorist.

Education: BSHE, Home Economics and English, Baylor University, Texas; BSN, University of Tennessee, Memphis; M.S., University of California, San Francisco; PhD New York University.

Service on Editorial boards: *Advances in Nursing Science, Nursing Science Quarterly, Journal of Prof. Nursing, Nursing Research* (Past), *Nursing and Health Care* (Past), *Western Journal of Nursing Research* (Past).

Previous Faculty Positions: University of Tennessee, New York University, The Pennsylvania State University.

Honors: Fellow, American Academy of Nursing, admitted 1976; *Who's Who in American Women*; Latin American Teaching Fellow; University of Tennessee, College of Nursing, Outstanding Alumnus Award; New York University, Division of Nursing, Distinguished Alumnus Award.

1

Origin of the Theory

Margaret Newman traced the origin of her theorizing on health to her prenursing days. As a young woman, Newman was influenced intuitively by her mother, who was diagnosed with amyotrophic lateral sclerosis. Newman (1986) noted while caring for her mother that although her mother was physically incapacitated, she was a whole person, viewed herself like any other person, and did not consider herself ill. Later, Newman formulated the premise that illness was part of health, and reflected the life pattern of a person. She arrived at this formulation through a synthesis of the knowledge gained in graduate study and her experiences with her mother. Newman claimed that nurses should recognize a person's life pattern and accept the pattern for what it means to that person. Newman first presented her theory at a Nurse Theorist Conference (1978). Newman (1979) first published her theory of health in a text titled *Theory Development in Nursing*. Her ideas were set forth in a chapter titled *Toward a Theory of Health*.

Newman credits nurse theorists, philosophers, and scholars with influencing her work. She was stimulated by discussions with Martha Rogers, who was one of her professors when she was a graduate student in nursing at New York University. Newman (1986) claims she was "intrigued and plagued" by Rogers's statement that "health and illness are simply expressions of the life process—one no more important than the other" (p. 4). She debated

3

with Rogers about this idea. After considerable thought, Newman
(1986) came to the realization that health and illness are a single
process. She likened this process to rhythmic phenomena, "manifest
in ups and downs, peaks and troughs, moving through varying
degrees of organization and disorganization, but all as one unitary
process" (p. 4). Newman (1986) formulated this unitary process of
health and illness into a concept that she called "pattern of the whole"
(p. 12). She referred to this pattern of the whole as expanding consciousness. Newman (1990a) claims that her theory of health as
expanding consciousness stems from Rogers's theory of unitary
human beings (Rogers, 1970). Rogers's assumption regarding the
patterning of persons in interaction with the environment is basic to
Newman's view that consciousness is a manifestation of an evolving
pattern of person-environment interaction.

Other scholars who influenced Newman in the development of
her theory of health were the biomedical engineer Itzhak Bentov
(1978), the philosopher Teilhard de Chardin (1959), the physicist
David Bohm (1980), the mathematician Arthur Young (1976a, 1976b),
and the physician Richard Moss (1981). Bentov's (1978) writing on
the evolution of consciousness provided Newman with logical
explanations for her earlier intuitive formulations. Teilhard de
Chardin's (1959) proposition that a person's consciousness continues to develop beyond the physical life and becomes a part of a
universal consciousness was congruent with Newman's view of
health as expanding consciousness. Bohm's (1980) theory of implicate order helped Newman to frame her theory of health into a
perspective of an underlying unseen pattern that manifests itself
in varying forms, including disease, and in the interconnectedness
and omnipresence of all that there is in life. Young's (1976a, 1976b)
theory of human evolution illuminated the critical importance of
pattern recognition or insight in the process of expanding consciousness (health). Young's theory provided Newman with the
impetus for the integration of her basic concepts of movement,
space, time, and consciousness into a dynamic portrayal of health
and life. Lastly, the description by Moss (1981) of love as the
highest level of consciousness provided Newman with an "affir-
mation and elaboration" of her "intuitions regarding the nature of
health" (Newman, 1986, pp. 5-6).

2

Assumptions of the Theory

Assumptions are statements accepted as given truths without proof. In order to use a theory, the assumptions must be accepted by the user. Assumptions set the foundation for the application of a particular theory.

Explicit Assumptions

An explicit assumption is a statement of truth that is fully and clearly expressed. The explicit assumptions of Newman's theory flow from her proposition that health is a synthesis of disease and nondisease. According to Newman (1979), the following assumptions are considered basic to her theory:

1. Health encompasses conditions heretofore described as illness, or in medical terms, pathology.
2. These pathological conditions can be considered a manifestation of the total pattern of the individual.
3. The pattern of the individual that eventually manifests itself as pathology is primary and exists prior to structural or functional changes.
4. Removal of the pathology in itself will not change the pattern of the individual.

5. If becoming "ill" is the only way an individual's pattern can manifest itself, then that is health for that person.
6. Health is the expansion of consciousness. (pp. 56-58)

Newman (1986) later regarded the sixth assumption as *the* theory, that is, *the* explanatory idea. It is this theory, the idea of health as expanding consciousness, that is elaborated by Newman.

Newman assumes that pattern is "an identification of the wholeness of the person" (Newman, 1990b, p. 132). Whatever manifests itself in a person's life is "an explication of the underlying pattern for that person" (Newman, 1990a, p. 38). Another assumption is that one's personal pattern is "part of a larger, undivided pattern of an expanding universe" (Newman, 1990a, pp. 38, 40). Basic to the understanding of Newman's theory of health is the assumption that one's personal "pattern is evolving unidirectionally ... toward a higher consciousness" (Newman, 1990b, p. 132).

Implicit Assumptions

Implicit assumptions are implied, rather than expressly stated, truths and are potentially contained or suggested in the descriptions of a theory. Implicit in Newman's theory are the two assumptions that humans are open energy systems, and that humans are in continual interconnectedness with a universe of open systems, frequently referred to as the environment. Another implicit assumption is that humans are continuously active in evolving their own pattern of the whole (health). A fourth implicit assumption is that humans are intuitive as well as cognitive and affective beings. This assumption is in tandem with the assumption that humans are capable of abstract thinking as well as sensation. There is also the implicit assumption that humans are more than the sum of their parts. Many of these assumptions were derived from Rogers's (1970) theory of unitary human beings.

3

Concepts of the Theory

Concepts are abstract ideas that provide a focus for thinking in a particular way. All theories have their own specific set of concepts that assist the student in understanding the meaning of the particular theory and its potential applications.

The basic concepts of Newman's theory of health are *consciousness, movement, space,* and *time.* Newman (1979) postulated that these concepts are interrelated in the following way:

1. Time and space have a complementary relationship.
2. Movement is a means by which space and time become a reality.
3. Movement is a reflection of consciousness.
4. Time is a function of movement.
5. Time is a measure of consciousness. (p. 60)

In addition to these four basic concepts, *pattern recognition, pattern,* and *expanding consciousness* are three concepts that are vital to the understanding of Newman's theory of health. These concepts are defined in the following paragraphs and are discussed in relation to the four paradigm concepts of nursing: *person, environment, health,* and *nursing* (Fawcett, 1989; Newman, 1983c).

Consciousness

Consciousness is defined by Newman (1986) as the

> informational capacity of the system: the capacity of the system to interact with its environment. In the human system, the informational capacity includes all of our present and developing knowledge about the nervous system, the endocrine system, the immune system, the genetic code, and so on. (p. 33)

Consciousness can be observed in the quality and diversity of interactions; the more complex the informational capacity and the more varied and more numerous the responses to the environment, the more highly developed is the human system.

Time-Space

Newman (1979) asserts that the world must be viewed as "a complicated network of interrelated changing events, as dynamic patterns of activity, with space aspects and time aspects" (p. 60). She insists that time and space are inextricably linked, yet one can identify aspects of each. For example, there is subjective time, objective time, time perspective, utilization of time, private time, coordinated time, and shared time. There is also personal space, inner space, territorial space, shared space, geographical and physical space, maneuverable space, distance regulating space, and life space (Newman, 1979, p. 61). Newman (1979) follows Bentov's (1978) lead in the study of subjective and objective time. Time perception, or the subjective sense of passing time, has been shown to vary with time of day, and is thought to be synchronized with other circadian rhythms, particularly body temperature. An increase in body temperature is related to the subjective sense of a greater amount of time passing than is revealed by clock time (objective time), and thus the feeling that time is dragging (Newman, 1986, p. 51).

The complementarity of time and space is viewed on different levels of analysis. Newman (1979, p. 61) uses an example from astronomy to illustrate the concept of the complementarity of time and space at the macrocosmic and microcosmic levels of systems analysis. That is, time flows in the opposite direction from human perspectives of time in the probability of antimatter galaxies, whereas with the possible existence of black holes in space, time and space are viewed as being wrapped up by gravitation in unimaginable ways. Subatomic particles of matter, at the microscopic level, appear to be going backward in time.

Newman (1979, 1982) has also shown through study how the complementarity of space and time can be seen in everyday events. The highly mobile individual lives in a world of expanded space and compartmentalized time. When a person's life space is decreased, as by either physical or social immobility, the person's time is increased. When physical or social life space is decreased, there is an opportunity for the person to focus attention on inner space. As a person focuses on the space within and transcends the limitations of three-dimensional space, the experience of time and the level of consciousness for that person are changed. Concepts of life space, personal space, and inner space can also be examined in relation to time, to show that the concepts of space and time are inextricably linked.

Movement

Newman (1979, p. 61) defines movement as the change occurring between two states of rest. It is an essential property of matter needed to bring about change. Without movement there is no manifest reality. Movement is the manifestation of consciousness and is the fundamental unit of analysis in Newman's theory of health. Movement represents "a pivotal choice point in the evolution of human consciousness" (Newman, 1986, p. 58). The task of the choice point is discovering new rules for living. Through movement, a person "discovers the world of time-space and establishes personal territory" (Newman, 1990a, p. 39). When persons no longer have the power of physical or social movement, they are forced to go beyond themselves. As persons "are able to recognize the boundarylessness and timelessness of human existence," they are free to return "to the ground of consciousness" (Newman, 1990a, p. 40). Movement is seen as an awareness of self, as a means of communicating, and as a daily mode of expression in gesture and speech.

To illustrate the manifestation of consciousness from the perspective of a person's movement, time, space, and environment
interactions, Newman (1986) cited several case examples of the
interaction patterns of women who were interviewed by graduate
students as part of a study of adult health. Two of these examples
are described below:

Case 1: Mrs. V. made repeated attempts to *move* away from her
husband and to *move* into an educational program to become more
independent. She felt she had no *space* for herself and she tried to
distance herself *(space)* from her husband. She felt she had no *time* for
leisure (self), was overworked, and was constantly meeting other
people's needs. She was submissive to the demands and criticisms
of her husband.

Case 2: Mrs. K. decreased her activities *(movement)* outside of home
(such as work and church) and appeared to be separating herself from
others (building up *space* around herself). Her husband was away
from home most of the time *(spatial distance)*. There were indications
that she was taking some form of sedatives or alcohol and slept most
of the time (altering *time*)(Newman, 1986, p. 56).

In applying her theory to these cases Newman (1986) explains:

> These examples reflect a diminished sense of self as reflected in
> contracted, almost nonexistent space-time dimension. They illustrate
> the relevance of the space time dimension in the sense of self. The
> point of intersection of the time, space, and movement dimensions
> represents the pattern of consciousness, the quality and quantity of
> interaction. In these examples the interaction . . . could be regarded
> as a low level of consciousness as defined by this model. (pp. 56-57)

It is at this juncture (pivotal point) that the nurse, in mutual
collaboration with both of these women, could act to facilitate their
expanding consciousness through pattern recognition and the discovery of new rules as the women move beyond the physical
restrictions of space and time.

Pattern Recognition

Pattern recognition is key in the process of evolving to higher
levels of consciousness. It occurs instantaneously and is the real-

ization of a truth, recognition of an insight, a principle, or an intuition (Newman, 1990a, p. 40). Insight has been "equated with the inner voice that some people consider their intuition" (Newman, 1986, p. 42). When pattern recognition occurs, it illuminates the possibilities for action. Newman (1990) uses a metaphor of being in the light or dark to describe the process of pattern recognition:

> It is like the difference between being in the dark and turning on the light: when the light comes on, one can see the possibilities for movement. Nursing facilitates this process by rhythmic connecting of the nurse with the client in an authentic way for the purpose of illuminating the pattern and discovering the new rules of a higher level of organization. (p. 40)

Pattern

Pattern is defined as relatedness, and is characterized by movement, diversity, and rhythm (Newman, 1986, p. 14). Pattern is intimately involved in energy exchange and transformation. Pattern is dynamic, in constant movement or change. The parts of pattern are diverse and are changing in relation to each other, and rhythm identifies the pattern. Pattern is recognized on the basis of variation in contrast, and may not be seen all at once. Pattern unfolds over time, with one configuration evolving into the next configuration and so forth. Pattern is manifest in the way one moves, the way one speaks and talks, and the way one relates with others. The pattern of the person can be identified across space and time. Pattern identifies the wholeness of the person (1986, p. 14; 1990a, p. 40; 1990b, p. 132).

Expanding Consciousness

Expanding consciousness is the evolving pattern of the whole. Expanding consciousness is health. It is the increasing complexity of the living system. Expanding consciousness is characterized by choice points, illuminations, and pattern recognition, resulting in a transformation and discovery of new rules of a higher organization (Newman, 1990a, p. 40).

4

Newman's Theory and Nursing's Paradigm Concepts

As Kuhn (1970) has noted, each discipline singles out certain phenomena with which it will deal in a unique manner. The concepts and propositions that identify and interrelate these phenomena comprise the paradigm of the discipline. Newman (1990b) uses the word *paradigm* to mean a worldview. The paradigm is the global perspective of a discipline and serves as a perspective from which the structure of the discipline develops.

Person, environment, health, and nursing are the four concepts that represent the basic components of nursing theory and are critical to the development of a paradigm for nursing (Fawcett, 1989; Newman, 1983b). According to Newman (1983c), "the domain of nursing has always included the nurse, the patient, the situation in which they find themselves, and the purpose of their being together, or the health of the patient" (p. 388).

The nursing theorists have placed different emphasis on each of the four basic concepts. *Person* has replaced *patient* as the concept used to represent humans. Humans are the "reason to be" for the discipline of nursing. This change in term from *patient* to *person* is reflective of the variety of settings within which nursing finds its practice domain. Newman (1979, 1986) has chosen to focus on health as the basic concept of nursing theory. In describing her theory, Newman explains person, environment, health, and nursing accordingly:

Person

Persons are dynamic patterns of energy and open systems in interaction with the environment. Persons are identified by their patterns of consciousness. The person does not possess consciousness. The person *is* consciousness (Newman, 1986, p. 33; 1990a, p. 40).

Environment

Environment is viewed as the event, situation, or phenomena with which an individual interacts. Environment is represented as a universe of open systems. The pattern of person-environment interaction constitutes health. These patterns of person-environment interaction are manifest in such observable phenomena as body temperature, pulse, and blood pressure; regimens of diet, rest, and exercise; neoplasms and biochemical variations; social relations and communications; cognition and emotions (Newman, 1986, p. 13).

A comprehensive portrayal of person-environment interactions can be gleaned from the nine dimensions of the North American Nursing Diagnostic Association (NANDA) assessment framework: exchanging, communicating, perceiving, relating, choosing, moving, valuing, feeling, and knowing (Kim & Moritz, 1982). These nine dimensions are defined and illustrated later in this book.

Health

Health is the expanding of consciousness. Health is constituted by the pattern of person-environment interaction. Health is *the evolving pattern of the whole of life.* (This is the crux of Newman's theory.) Health is the synthesis of disease/nondisease. Health is the process of transformation to higher levels of consciousness (Newman, 1979, 1986).

Nursing

Newman (1986) identified the critical task for gaining an understanding of her theory of health as the ability to view the concepts of movement-space-time in relation to each other, simultaneously, as patterns of expanding consciousness. She sees the goal of nursing as one of assisting "people to utilize the power that is within them as they evolve toward higher levels of consciousness" (Newman, 1979, p. 67). Nursing practice, according to Newman, "is directed toward recognizing the pattern of the person in interaction with the environment and accepting it as a process of evolving consciousness" (Newman, 1986, p. 88). Nursing facilitates the process of pattern recognition by a "rhythmic connecting of the nurse with the client in an authentic way for the purpose of illuminating the pattern and discovering the new rules of a higher level of organization" (Newman, 1990a, p. 40).

Newman (1986) calls for nursing to employ a partnership model of non-intervention. She describes this relationship:

> The professional enters into a partnership with the client with the mutual goal of participating in an authentic relationship, trusting that in the process of its evolving, both will grow and become healthier in the sense of higher levels of consciousness. (p. 68)

According to Newman (1990b), "people need a partner" in the process of expanding consciousness," particularly when they are suffering and do not find any meaning in what is going on" (p. 136). Mutuality is key to the nurse-client partner relationship. Mutuality between nurse and client occurs in the process of the nurse's assisting the client in making and implementing the choices that emerge through pattern recognition (Newman, 1990b). The nurse connects with a client when the client is faced with a situation that she or he does not know how to handle. Or, when he or she is searching for new rules, when old rules for living no longer work. The nurse releases the desire to control the situation, interacts with the client, shares his or her consciousness, and helps to identify the pattern that is manifest. The task of the nurse is to be free of a predetermined agenda, to be present with the client as the possibilities for transformation emerge, and to support the client as she or he makes decisions and choices (Newman, 1990b, pp. 136-137).

5

Propositions

Propositions are ideas brought forward for consideration, acceptance, or adoption. They are declarations of the design or intention of a theory. They~are statements of truth to be demonstrated or operations to be performed.

The fundamental proposition in Newman's model is the view that health and illness are synthesized as health. In this proposition, Newman (1979, 1986) applies Hegelian dialectical logic; that is, "that thought proceeds by contradiction and the recognition of contradiction, the overall pattern being one of thesis, antithesis and synthesis" (Flew, 1984, p. 94). Newman proposes that one state of being (disease) unites with its opposite (nondisease) resulting in a synthesis of the two. The fusion of these two antithetical concepts brings forth a synthesis that can be regarded as health (Newman, 1979, p. 56).

The proposition that health is to be viewed as an evolving pattern of the whole is basic to the understanding of Newman's theory of health. Newman (1986) explains:

> The emerging paradigm of health is pattern recognition. It involves moving from looking at parts to looking at patterns. The pattern is information that depicts the whole, understanding of the meaning of all the relationships at once. It is a fundamental attribute of all there is and gives unity in diversity. (p. 13)

15

This conceptualization of health as pattern also finds root in Rogers's (1970) theory of unitary man. Rogers's insistence that health and illness are simply manifestations of the rhythmic fluctuations of the life process led Newman to the view that health and illness are a unitary process moving through variations in order-disorder. From this perspective it is no longer possible to view health as a continuum extending from illness to wellness. The illness-wellness continuum is part of the worldview of health as the absence of disease, because as one moves toward the wellness end of the continuum, one moves away from disease by either preventing the disease or promoting behaviors that are thought to promote health (Newman, 1990b). According to Newman's view, health encompasses disease as a meaningful aspect of health. In this view then, health and the evolving pattern of consciousness are one and the same (1990a).

6

Overview of Newman's Theory

Newman (1979, 1986) posits that health is process. She claims that pattern is the essence of a holistic view of health. In this view, health is the flow of life. It is a kaleidoscopic evolution of patterning, with contradictions, ambiguities, and paradoxes, continually synthesized into insights that lead to an ever-expanding consciousness (transformation). Movement is fundamental to this dialectical process of transformation. Pattern recognition is a spontaneous insight in relation to a shift in organizational complexity, affording greater freedom and variety of responses to any given situation. Expanding consciousness occurs as a process of pattern recognition (insights) following a synthesis of contradictory events or disturbances in the flow of daily living. Disease and nondisease serve as reflections of a larger whole. The proposition that health is the synthesis of disease and nondisease is a revolutionary way of conceptualizing health.

Newman (1986; 1990a, p. 39) describes the parallels between her theory of health as expanding consciousness and Young's (1976b) theory of the evolution of consciousness. For instance, Young claims that humans enter this world with a state of potential freedom and move through several stages of loss of degrees of freedom as they descend into a deterministic physical world. Young calls his first stage the stage of binding. In the binding stage, a person is bound into the larger network of the whole in which everything is regulated, and the individual is sacrificed for the good of the whole. There is very little individual identity or choice in the binding stage. The binding stage is followed by the centering stage, whereby a person establishes an identity, self-consciousness, and self-determination. In this centering stage, the self breaks with the authority of the binding stage. The centering stage is a competitive, persuasive stage in which a person seeks to gain power over others and gain power for him- or herself. The turning point is the stage called choice. In this stage, the things that worked in the past no longer work. What was formerly considered progress is no longer seen as progress. It is in the choice stage that the individual must master the task of learning new rules. Reformation or transformation is preceded by a realization of self-limitation. It is this realization that makes it possible for persons to begin the evolution back to freedom by going beyond themselves and entering into the stages of decentering and unbinding.

Newman (1990a) illustrates the similarity between her theory of health as expanding consciousness and Young's (1976b) evolving consciousness theory, as shown in Figure 6.1.

According to Newman (1990a):

A person comes into being from the ground of consciousness and loses freedom as one is bound in time and finds one's identity in space. Matters of time-space are very much involved in one's struggles for self-determination and status. Movement represents the choice point. It is central to understanding the nature of reality. Through movement one discovers the world of time-space and establishes personal territory. It is also when movement is restricted that one becomes aware of personal limitations and the fact that the old rules don't work anymore. When one no longer has the power of movement (either physical or social), it is necessary to go beyond oneself. As one is able to recognize the boundarylessness and timelessness of human existence, one gains the freedom of returning to the ground of consciousness. (pp. 39-40)

To illustrate this process, Newman (1986) describes the restrictions of her own mobility and her transformation in terms of space and time during her experience as primary caregiver for her mother, who was incapacitated with amyotrophic lateral sclerosis. Not only was Newman's mother not free to move about in space or to control her own time, but these restrictions also applied to Newman.

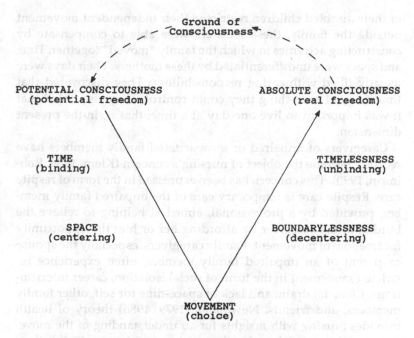

Figure 6.1. Parallel Between Newman's Theory of Expanding Consciousness and Young's Stages of Human Evolution

SOURCE: Adapted from Newman, Margaret A. (1990). Newman's theory of health as praxis. *Nursing Science Quarterly, 3*(1), 39. Reprinted with permission from Chestnut House Publications, © 1990.

The freedom to come and go as and when she chose was no longer an option. Usually taken for granted, these mobility options are altered by situations and circumstances that render imprudent or impossible the freedom of movement. According to Newman (1986), restrictions of movement force a person into a realm beyond space and time. The old rules for relating no longer work. Persons find themselves faced with their selves and their own inner resources. They are confronted with the quality of their relationships and their ability to live in the present. Given these circumstances, the developmental task involves becoming open to the transformation, allowing it to occur as the person transcends space and time and moves to higher consciousness.

West (1984) observed this process in mothers of developmentally disabled children. Even though the mothers' care responsibilities

of their disabled children restricted their independent movement
outside the family, these mothers were able to compensate by
constructing activities in which the family "moved" together. Time
and space were undifferentiated by these mothers. Their days were
usually filled with caring responsibilities. They discovered that
time was not something they could control. They also noted that
it was important to live one day at a time, that is, in the present
dimension.

Caregivers of impaired or incapacitated family members have
recently become the object of nursing's concern (Klein, 1989; Robinson, 1990). This concern has been expressed in the form of respite
care. Respite care is temporary care of the impaired family member, provided by a professional, aimed at helping to relieve the
burden of the caregiver by affording her or him the opportunity
for freedom of movement. Family caregivers, especially the spouse
or parent of an impaired family member, often experience restricted movement in the form of social isolation, career interrup-
tions, financial drain, and lack of space-time for self, other family
members, and friends. Newman's (1979, 1986) theory of health
provides nursing with insights for an understanding of the movement restrictions of these family caregivers, and suggests directions
for assisting them in finding new rules for living and transcending
their movement restrictions.

7

Evolving the Pattern of the Whole

Newman (1987) claims that pattern recognition comes from within
the observer, which means that with any set of data or sequence of
events, "an infinite number of patterns are possible" (p. 38). Patterns unfold in time and cannot be predicted with certainty, because the additional information has not happened yet. The evolving
pattern of the person is best portrayed as sequential patterns over
time. To illustrate a person's pattern of the whole, Newman (1987)
described a case of a client experiencing a crisis event. The example
was obtained from the caseload of a community health nursing
colleague. The analysis of the unfolding pattern is portrayed in
three time frames: prior to the crisis, immediately following the
crisis event, and fifteen weeks after the crisis.

A Case Study: Client K

This is the description of client K's pattern: She was a young
divorced woman who was solely responsible for the care of her
two preschool-age children. K's means of support was generated
through her provision of day care for three other preschool children and an infant. The event that brought K to the attention of the
nurse was the sudden death of the infant while K was caring for
him in her home. Shortly after the infant's death, the nurse contacted

21

the client and offered information about Sudden Infant Death Syndrome (SIDS). The client asked for help in relating to her own two children, aged two and five, who had witnessed the event and who had since manifested behavior changes. When the nurse visited the home, she found it in complete disarray. The children were fighting with each other and their mother. K complained of insomnia, fatigue, and loss of interest in her children. She was tearful and expressed a desire to be alone. The nurse provided suggestions for immediate action in relation to the children, and was instrumental in steering K toward a SIDS support group. K later reported that she had received considerable comfort as a result of her attendance at the support group meetings.

The nurse maintained periodic contact with K. On visiting the home fifteen weeks after the SIDS event, the nurse found that, although K was still sad about the infant's death, she had begun to reach out (move) to others in her family and in the community. She had obtained an instructor's license in cardiopulmonary resuscitation (CPR) and was already teaching a CPR class. K volunteered to serve on a local health service board. She helped to present a program about SIDS for day-care providers, made contact with babysitters who had had similar experiences with SIDS, and arranged for the distribution of printed information about SIDS to licensed day-care providers.

Prior to the SIDS event, K was feeling bored with her life. She was relatively isolated from adult interactions. Contacts with her ex-husband were limited, and she was not close to her family of origin, even though her mother and brother lived nearby. At the time the nurse entered the situation, K's pattern of interaction could be described as one of disorganization. She expressed feelings of sadness and guilt related to the infant death and was frustrated with her child-care responsibilities. As she moved to a new level of consciousness through a synthesis of the SIDS experience and her interactions with the nurse and the SIDS support group, she was able to develop a new set of rules for living. For the first time, she was able to reach out for assistance to her mother-in-law, who began to participate with her in the care of the children. She reported that she had maintained a friendship with the parents of the infant who died suddenly. She encouraged her children to openly discuss the experience of the infant's death and to ask questions freely. K also expressed the feeling that she had

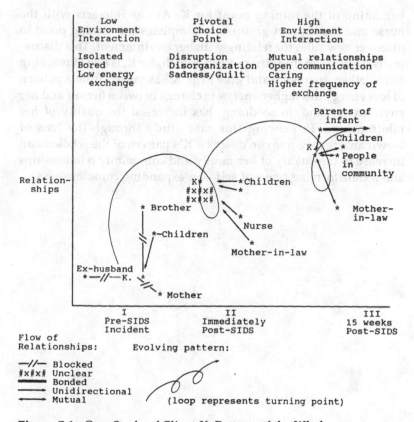

Figure 7.1. Case Study of Client K: Pattern of the Whole.

SOURCE: Adapted from Newman, M. (1984). Patterning. In M. Duffy & N. Pender (Eds.), *Conceptual issues in health promotion: Report of proceedings of a wingspread conference* (p. 40). Indianapolis: Sigma Theta Tau. Reprinted by permission.

become more outgoing and caring in her relationships with other people.

A diagram of three sequential patterns from client K's life can be seen in Figure 7.1.

The first pattern is seen as a relatively closed space-time, low-energy system in which K existed, almost entirely alone, with the young children in her life. Immediately following the death of the infant, her pattern is marked by disruption and disorganization. K begins to move through the events and confronts her feelings and the children's behavior changes. This period can be viewed as a beginning of the turning point for K. As she interacts with the nurse and the support group, she completes the turning point to discover new rules for relating with her environment. This discovery is depicted in the third pattern, which, for K, is one of reaching out to others to receive and give help. K has moved from a pattern of low energy to a higher energy exchange between herself and her environment and, in so doing, has increased the quality of her relationships. In viewing this case study through the lens of Newman's theory, one can describe K's pattern of the whole as an increase in the quality of her family and community relationships and a transforming sense of self—an expanding consciousness.

8

Framework for Assessing the Pattern of the Whole

Newman (1986, 1987) has suggested that the assessment framework developed by nurse theorists for the North American Nursing Diagnostic Association (NANDA) can be used in initial efforts to identify pattern of the whole. Manifestations of the unitary pattern are expressed in the dimensions of the NANDA framework: exchanging, communicating, valuing, relating, choosing, moving, perceiving, feeling, and knowing.

Newman (1986, p. 74) has defined these nine assessment dimensions relative to her theory of health, as modified from those accepted by the nurse theorist group at the third and fourth conferences of NANDA (Kim & Moritz, 1982). Exchanging involves the interchange of energy and matter between person and environment. It also involves the transformation of energy from one form to another. Communicating involves the interchange of information from one system to another. Relating is the process of connecting with other persons and with the environment. Valuing is the process of assigning worth. Choosing involves the selection of one or more alternatives. Moving is the process of rhythmic alternating between activity and rest. Perceiving is the process of receiving and interpreting information. Feeling involves a sensing of physical and intuitive awareness. Knowing is the process of personal recognition of self and world.

The process of assessing the pattern of the whole proceeds in the following fashion: The nurse surveys the client-environment interaction data in terms of the nine assessment dimensions, describes a nonjudgmental pattern of interaction, and searches for the underlying pattern of the whole. A case study illustrating this assessment process can be found in Newman's 1984 *American Journal of Nursing* article. A description of the case study assessment data, gathered from the client, using the NANDA framework, and interpreted from the perspective of Newman's theory, is included here.

A Case Study: Client X

Ms. X is 40 years old and is the youngest of five sisters. She is currently on a leave of absence from a recently acquired secretarial job due to right arm and right breast edema that interfered with her ability to work. She is 20 pounds overweight and does not engage in any routine exercise or recreation, even though she had formerly been a dancing instructor. She reverses the few decisions her husband makes and speaks angrily about him, describing him as a passive, incompetent person who is incapable of decision making. It is unclear to what extent she communicates this perception and anger to her husband. She says he is the only kind of man that she could live with because he provides her with the freedom to act alone and to do what she wants.

She speaks little of her two sons, who are 12 and 14 years of age. When she does mention them, her comments are also filled with criticism. Ms. X also describes her father, who is now dead, as a passive and invisible person.

Ms. X lost her mother to multiple myeloma. Ms. X was her mother's sole care provider during the last three months of her illness. She speaks frequently of her mother.

She views her nuclear family as totally dependent on her and presents herself as a martyr. For instance, she must take care of the house, clothing, and cooking with little assistance from her sons and husband.

She claims she is fatigued and has difficulty sleeping, suppressing her problems during the day and awakening during the night to ponder them. She has designated Saturday mornings as her private space-time, and prohibits any intrusions. She indicates that she does not have friends. She makes phone visits with her sisters, but they are geographically distant. Her nieces have come to assist her during previous illnesses.

Her boss describes her as a creative, self-directive, and capable woman, who appears engrossed and stoic, yet tense beneath the surface. Outside the work setting, she does not associate with coworkers, although at work she is sensitive to their needs.

She has had two previous hospital admissions. Once, at age 20, she was admitted for dysmenorrhea, diagnosed with endometriosis, and told that she would be unable to conceive children. She had no trouble conceiving her two sons. She was hospitalized for a possible hysterectomy at age 36, but was found to have a right ovarian cyst. A right oophorectomy was performed instead. Following this surgery, she continued to experience painful dysmenorrhea and irregular periods. She disagreed with the surgeon's claim that it was not necessary to do the hysterectomy, and was very distressed that it was not done.

According to Newman (1984), the data obtained from clients tend to cluster within two or three dimensions of the NANDA schema. The experienced nurse may identify the emerging pattern without collecting data in every dimension of the assessment framework. Even though many aspects of the life pattern of Ms. X are unknown, the experienced nurse may begin to visualize the emerging pattern (nursing diagnosis) even with only the sparsest of data. Newman (1984) identified the emerging pattern for Ms. X: retention of energy, characterized by trapped fluid in the right arm and breast, excess fat, and anger and self-pity; repulsion and control of others, characterized by criticism, distancing, and self sacrifice; and internal conflict with minimal channels for expression.

A more detailed account of this case can be seen in Table 8.1 (developed by Newman, 1982), depicting specific observations and organized according to the nine assessment dimensions described above. The assessment framework, based on a unitary pattern of person-environment interactions, provides a holistic approach toward nursing diagnosis. Ms. X's hospitalization may be viewed as a choice point. The task Ms. X is now facing is how to discover new rules for engaging in meaningful, reciprocal relationships. She may not know how. This is where the nurse, through a mutual negotiation with the client, may help her to get in touch with her pattern of blocked energy. Through a process of mutual

TABLE 8.1 The Emerging Pattern of Ms. X

Dimension	Observation	Emerging Pattern
Exchanging	History of endometriosis. Right oophorectomy, cyst removal. Overweight 20 pounds. Trapped fluid in right arm and breast.	Retention.
Communicating	Directive, corrective, and critical communication with husband and sons. Maintains distance with co-workers with only business level interactions.	Repels outflow, distancing via space and time, building tension with no outlet.
Relating	Subordinate relationship to boss, dominant relationship to husband and sons, unclear relationship with sisters. No friends. Previous commitment to mother. Disregard of husband and father. Distances self from family.	Vertical relationships with distancing; bonding more easily with women than with men.
Valuing	Being alone. Doing what she wants to do. Being in control. Doing a good job.	Centered on self.
Choosing	To assume full responsibility for care of mother. To stay married to a man whom she does not respect. To work in subordinate role. To make family decisions on her own.	Unilateral. Apparently without any consideration of the alternatives.
Moving	Performs household tasks. Moved to sedentary job from job of dance teacher. Fatigued—insomnia. Arm restricted, can't do job.	Restricted. Diminished.
Perceiving	Sees husband as incompetent, physician as wrong, sisters as uncaring, self as responsible, and self-sacrificing.	Selective, self-centered.

continued

TABLE 8.1 Continued

Dimension	Observation	Emerging Pattern
Feeling	Fatigue. Edema discomfort. Appears tense underneath calm. Dissatisfied, angry with regard to family relationships. Absence of self-regard. Previous dysmenorrhea.	Internal unrest.
Knowing	Recollects mother's illness and death. Suppresses concerns during day, tries to think them through at night. Knows something is wrong physically. Knows how to meet other people's needs but little about herself.	Internal turmoil. Lack of clarity regarding self.

NOTE: Newman no longer uses a table format to represent patterning of the whole. Adapted from: Newman, M. (1984). Nursing diagnosis: Looking at the whole. *American Journal of Nursing, 84*(12), 1496-1499. Copyright by American Journal of Nursing. Reprinted by permission.

authentic relating, the nurse can facilitate the insight, the discovery of new rules for living, and the empowerment Ms. X needs to transform her emerging pattern into an evolving of health as expanding consciousness (Newman, 1984).

Practitioners in clinical settings may find the case of Ms. X useful in applying and interpreting the NANDA framework as Newman has defined it. However, it is necessary to note that the table in the 1982 *American Journal of Nursing* article was one of Newman's earliest attempts to illustrate a clinical example of the NANDA assessment framework relative to the identification of pattern. She has now revised her thinking on the use of this table illustration and claims that a better way to represent the emerging pattern of the whole is to record the development of sequential patterns over time (as seen in Figure 7.1). Table 8.1, depicting data from client X, fails to show the pattern in sequence. In critique of Table 8.1, Newman notes that the table combines information nonsequentially, from different phases of Ms. X's life, and, as such, does not reveal the emerging pattern. She claims that the organization of data in this way implies a more mechanical method of determining pattern than is actually the case. Her current thinking on pattern depiction is to organize data in a narrative form and let the pattern "fall out" from the data (Newman, 1991, June 11; July 4, personal communications).

It may be of interest to students of nursing theory to see that the task of pattern identification/recognition is still being worked out by Newman. The 1982 journal article, chronicling the case study of Ms. X, as illustrated in Table 8.1, serves as a beginning point in the evolution of Newman's thinking on this task. She continues to work out better ways to discover this process of pattern recognition and to illustrate the emerging pattern of the whole.

Kalb (1990) applied Newman's theory of health and the pattern recognition model in a program of care developed with high-risk pregnant women who were hospitalized with adverse physiological manifestations of maternal-fetal health. For these women, their high-risk pregnancy represented a critical event that yielded alterations in their physical and social world. The alterations in each woman's pattern of health required energy from the environment to produce a higher level of organization and a new level of consciousness. Through the intervention of pattern recognition, Kalb (1990) claimed, the nurses caring for these women with high-risk pregnancy provided a source of the environmental energy.

Kalb (1990) portrayed the manifestations of pattern in pregnancy using, as her framework, the four concepts of Newman's theory of health: movement, time, space, and consciousness. The alterations created by pregnancy include changes in a woman's pattern of movement. Pregnant women move more slowly. The pregnant woman's perceptions are altered by hormonal changes that lead to feelings of fatigue. These feelings of fatigue may have significant effects on the woman's ability to continue her previous pattern of interaction with the environment and the control she has previously been able to maintain in the quality of her interactions. A woman's perceptions of her own rhythmicity and movement may be altered by the awareness of her unborn child's pattern of activity and movement, as well as the circadian pattern of the woman's uterine activity and contractions.

The pregnant woman's perception of time is frequently altered as she anticipates the birth of her child. Time seems to drag, especially in the third trimester, when movement is slowed and fatigue is increased. Personal tempo and time experience of the pregnant women may follow the basic rhythm or pattern used throughout the woman's life experiences, and are linked to space and movement.

As the pregnancy continues and the unborn child develops, the woman's size and shape are altered and become larger. This increased body space frequently results in an altered self-image. It is also interesting to consider the space-time-movement laden language used in describing a woman's pregnancy. Movement-space-time connotations are exemplified: for example, in the phrase "expected date of confinement." The notion of restricted movement and the perceptions of altered space-time during the experience of pregnancy are images explicitly created by our language (Kalb, 1990).

The awareness of new sensations within the pregnant woman's body, the feelings of fetal movement, the hormonal fluctuations, the alterations of her own bodily rhythms, and the synchronicity of self with the unborn child are all manifestations of an altered pattern of consciousness. Alterations in patterns of interaction with her partner, significant others, and in her internal and external environment are also critical attributes of consciousness in the woman's evolving pattern of pregnancy.

Pregnant women who are hospitalized for high-risk complications also experience changing patterns of movement, space, and time. Movement is restricted to bed or within the room, nursing unit, or hospital, and may be further limited by the length of an intravenous tubing. Time becomes routinized according to the hospital schedule, as in prescribed times for visitors, vital signs, meals, grooming, nursing shift changes, and so on. The woman's typical routine, such as having baby showers, attending childbirth classes, and preparing a room for the baby, are frequently suspended during her hospital confinement. In the hospital, the pregnant woman must share space with nonsignificant others; is confined in an unfamiliar environment; separated from her partner, family, and friends; and is often forced to spend time alone or interacting with strangers. Her perceptions of space are often altered by the viewpoint of always being in a reclining or sitting position. Her awareness is shifted abruptly to self and to the unborn child's well-being. As the woman's perceptions of movement, time, and space are altered in the management of her high-risk pregnancy, her capacity to interact with her environment changes, thus indicating changes in her level of consciousness.

Kalb (1990) described a Minnesota hospital program, based on the concept of pattern recognition, designed for high-risk women to actively participate in the monitoring and management of their preterm labor. The women, in partnership with a nurse, learn to recognize and identify the physical manifestations of pregnancy that they are experiencing, and to integrate the characteristics of their experiences into their pattern of the whole. They are taught to keep a diary of self-palpations of uterine activity and contractions and pulse rates. Based on this record, the women are taught to self-administer subcutaneous drug therapy (terbutaline, a tocolytic medication) for labor control. The client, as "partner with the nurse and active participant in the experience of managing her high-risk pregnancy, is able to recognize and describe her pattern of the whole" (Kalb, 1990, p. 179). Therefore, the client with a high-risk pregnancy responds more fully in synchrony with her own pattern.

Recently, Newman, Lamb, and Michaels (1991) selected Carondelet Health Center, Tuscon, Arizona, as their demonstration site to show how Newman's theory of health applies to nursing care delivery in the new nursing role of the case manager. These authors recommend the blending of theory and practice as an initial step toward defining and documenting the nursing practice needed to satisfy third-party payers. The bibliography contains other examples of applications of Newman's theory in clinical settings.

9

Newman's Theory and Family Health

Newman (1983b) extended her theory of health as expanding consciousness to explain the health of the family. According to Newman, family health is the expansion of consciousness of the family. Consciousness for the family system is the increase in the quantity and quality of responses of the family members manifested in greater spontaneity within the family. The spontaneous interactive pattern of the family, expressed through movement, is seen as a manifestation of expanding consciousness.

Family space, time, and movement dimensions have been reconceptualized in terms of the family. Family applications of Newman's theory of health can be found in a chapter by Marchione (1986b) in Winstead Fry's edited text titled *Case Studies in Nursing Theory*. A community application is also described by Marchione (1986a) in her supplemental chapter to the Newman (1986) text.

10

Research and Newman's Theory

Newman's (1966) earliest research effort was qualitative in nature, based on individualized, reciprocal interaction with hospitalized patients, and it incorporated her thoughts and feelings as factors that made a difference in the findings. Newman intended to identify needs of patients (content), but in the course of doing so, the more significant finding was the process used in identifying the needs. That particular study "contributed directly to the knowledge of nursing practice," and Newman (1990a) claims, "it was also personally meaningful [to her] as the investigator" as well as "to the patients who participated as subjects" (p. 37).

Later, Newman (1972, 1976) converted holistic parameters of a person's living experience into manipulable artifacts in the laboratory in an attempt to test several very basic relationships of movement, time, and consciousness. The outcomes of these studies were tangential to the meaningful experiences that were their source. The aspect of her research that stimulated insight regarding the relevance to nursing practice was the debriefing interviews in which Newman sought a greater understanding of the person's experiences in movement-time-space. She continued to pursue this line of investigation in an attempt to demonstrate the expansion of consciousness with age (Newman, 1982; Newman & Gaudiano, 1984). She claims her inability in these studies to adequately capture the major variables or to rule out intervening variables raised questions regarding the validity of the methods to test the theory, and pointed her toward other modes of inquiry. Gradually, she moved to a method of inquiry that was consistent with her theoretical assumptions; that is, the open, interactive nature of the evolving pattern. She concluded that the important part of her research was the process involved in interacting with patients. Newman (1990a) asserts that "the *process* in nursing, and in nursing research, *is* the *content*" (p. 38).

Newman (1983a) proposes that pattern recognition is the appropriate method for nursing research. In an editorial to the readers of *Advances in Nursing Science*, she calls for nurse researchers to use the method of pattern in the development of nursing knowledge.

Schorr, Farnahm, and Ervin (1991) used Newman's theory of health as expanding consciousness in their study of the phenomenon of powerlessness among aging women. Using a survey design and quantitative analysis, they sought to identify a pattern of relationships among the impact of chronic illness, frame of temporal reference, death anxiety, hopelessness, and powerlessness. Among their sample of sixty women, ranging in age from 65 to 93 years, they found that a majority of the women manifested high levels of perceived situational control or powerfulness. The majority of their subjects, using their chronic illnesses, diminished functional ability, and decreased control over daily activities as choice points, synthesized this situation into a pattern of powerfulness and hopefulness for the future. It was not stated whether the clients in this study synthesized their choice points as a result of their partnerships with a nurse or whether the synthesis occurred independently. The authors interpreted their findings of powerfulness and hopefulness patterns in aging women as reflections of expanding consciousness and awareness of health as the pattern of the whole (Schorr, Farnahm, & Ervin, 1991, p. 62).

Recently, Newman (1990a) described the elements of a qualitative praxis research method that are necessary to elaborate the pattern of a person's expanding consciousness. These elements are: (a) establishing the mutuality of the process of inquiry; (b) focusing on the most meaningful persons and events in the interviewee's life; (c) organizing the data in narrative form and displaying it as sequential patterns over time; and (d) a sharing of the interviewer's perception of the pattern with the interviewee and seeking revision or confirmation.

According to Newman (1990a), in praxis research the interviewees gain insight into their own pattern and concomitant illumination of their action possibilities. These insights and illuminations are inherent in the research process. Praxis research requires negotiation, reciprocity, and empowerment. Praxis research requires a mutual relationship between interviewee and researcher. These are the characteristics of praxis whereby research, practice, and theory are inseparable.

Moch's (1990) study is one example of the use of praxis research. Her research was designed for the purpose of describing and explaining the manifestation of health in illness. She collaborated with 20 women, ranging in age from 38 to 60 years, who had experienced breast cancer. The women were asked to describe their experiences with breast cancer through two open-ended interviews. Patterns of their person-environment interaction were identified by extracting themes from the interview data. Changes in their relatedness to others and to the environment were apparent as a predominant theme. The women experienced increasing richness in their relatedness to others. They were increasingly receptive to and felt closer to others, particularly members of their family; they were more open to experiencing others' expressions of caring. As they became aware of their own mortality, they found new meaning and value in their lives. They were more open to their surroundings and experienced greater enjoyment in life. These manifestations of the increasing quality and diversity of their lives are examples of their expanding consciousness in the experience of breast cancer.

Regardless of the level of disease or disability of given persons, the action potential of their patterns of interaction focus on their relationships with other people. The task they are facing is how to engage in meaningful, reciprocal relationships through the discovery of new rules. They want to talk about things that are important to them, to express a full range of emotions, and to be truly themselves. But often they do not know how. According to Newman (1990a), it is at this point that nursing, using praxis research, comes into the picture. Praxis research involves a mutuality between researcher and interviewee. This research method is an embodiment of negotiation, reciprocity, and empowerment. Through praxis research nurses can assist people in discovering the new rules and in recognizing the action potential of the pattern, thus opening the way for transformation and for the unfolding of a higher level of consciousness. Praxis research intertwines theory, practice, and research. As Lather (1986) has explained, in praxis research there must be an intersection between people's self-understanding and the researcher's theoretical stance, which seeks to provide a change-enhancing context. The praxis researcher seeks theory that grows out of context-embedded data. Nurse researchers are urged to use praxis research to help participants understand and change their situations. Newman's theory of health as expanding consciousness is conducive to the method of praxis research (Newman, 1990a).

Newman and Moch (in press) applied praxis research, explicating Newman's theory of health, in a recent study of person-environment patterns of eleven people with coronary heart disease (CHD). The study emphasized the meaning of the disruption that CHD represented for each person. Narratives of evolving patterns of meaning based on the clients' descriptions were later confirmed or revised by the clients. Similarities in meaningful patterns described by the clients who participated in the study were: (a) a sense of who they were; (b) a need to develop better relationships with members of their family; and (c) the desire to discover new ways of living.

The mutual process of pattern recognition in this study was seen as a rhythmic coming together and moving apart of client and nurse in a shared consciousness until the client was able to see clearly and take action to express her/his meaning. This method of cooperative inquiry was recommended as a model for nursing research and practice.

11

Conclusion

In this book, the Newman theory of health as expanding consciousness has been explained. Major propositions, assumptions, and concepts of the theory have been identified, described, and defined. Case studies have been included to illustrate the application of the theory in practice. Research applications by Newman and others have been noted. Newman's praxis research method has been explicated.

Newman's theory of health can be useful as a guide for nursing practice and research. The praxis research method identified by Newman has begun to take hold in academic and practice settings. According to Newman (1990a), current research focuses on the unfolding pattern of person-environment over time and incorporates the authentic involvement of the nurse researcher as a participant with the client in the process of expanding consciousness.

Newman's (1986) book on the theory of health as expanding consciousness has been critiqued by Watson (1987), Cowling (1988), Pearson (1988), Silva (1988), and Smith (1990). Newman's theory of health as praxis research has been critiqued by Boyd (1990), Ray (1990), and Batey (1991). Readers are encouraged to study the original writings of Newman and the critiques of her works for a complete understanding of this revolutionary theory of health.

Glossary

Consciousness

Consciousness is the informational capacity of the system (individual, family, or community). It is the ability of the system to interact with the environment. Consciousness includes cognitive and affective awareness, and the interconnectedness of the entire living system, which includes growth processes and physiochemical maintenance as well as the immune system, the genetic code, the nervous system, and so on. Consciousness is an indivisible pattern of information that is part of a larger undivided pattern of an expanding universe (Newman, 1986, p. 33; 1990a, p. 38).

Environment

Environment is represented as a universe of open systems. Environment is an energy field, and is viewed as the event, situation, or phenomena with which an individual interacts. The pattern of environment-person interaction constitutes health. Manifestations of the environment-person interaction are seen in such observable phenomena as body temperature, pulse, and blood pressure; neoplasms and biochemical variations; regimens of diet, rest, and exercise; social relations, communications, cognition, and emotions (Newman, 1986, p. 13). A comprehensive portrayal of patterns of person-environment interaction can be viewed through the nine assessment dimensions of the North American Nursing Diagnosis Association framework; that is, exchanging, communicating, valuing, relating, choosing, moving, perceiving, feeling, and knowing (Kim & Moritz, 1982). In this glossary these terms are defined separately under the concept NANDA Assessment Framework.

Expanding Consciousness
Expanding consciousness is the evolving pattern of the whole. Expanding consciousness is the increasing complexity of the living system. Expanding consciousness is characterized by a choice point, an illumination, and pattern recognition, resulting in a transformation and discovery of new rules of a higher level of organization. Expanding consciousness is health (Newman, 1990a, p. 40).

Health
Health is the expanding of consciousness. Health is the evolving pattern of the whole of life. (This is the crux of Newman's theory.) Health is a synthesis of disease-non-disease. Health is the process of transformation to higher levels of consciousness (Newman, 1979, p. 58; 1990a, p.40).

Hegelian Dialectical Logic
Dialectic is a term derived from the Greek word that means to converse or to discourse. The dialectic that is ascribed to the Greek philosopher Socrates is close to this sense. It refers to his conversational method of argument, involving thought as question and answer. Hegel, a late eighteenth and early nineteenth century philosoper, described a pattern of dialectical logic that thought must follow. Hegel argued that thought proceeds by contradiction and the reconciliation of contradiction. This dialectical logic and overall pattern of thought is one of thesis, antithesis, and synthesis. For Hegel, thought is reality, and the laws that thought must follow are also the laws that govern reality (Flew, 1984, p. 94).

Movement
Movement is the change occurring between two states of rest. It is an essential property of matter needed to bring about change. Movement represents the choice point in transcending physical determinism. Movement is central to understanding the nature of reality. Movement is a manifestation of consciousness. Movement is an awareness of self and a means of communicating (Newman, 1979, pp. 61-63; 1990a, p. 39).

NANDA Assessment Framework
Nurse theorists developed a framework for the North American Nursing Diagnostic Association (NANDA) by delineating nine assessment dimensions for use in nursing diagnosis (Kim & Moritz, 1982). Manifestations of unitary pattern are expressed in the nine dimensions of the NANDA framework. Newman (1986) has recommended that the NANDA assessment framework be used in initial efforts to identify pattern of the whole, and has specifically defined these nine assessment dimensions relative to her theory of health:

Choosing. Choosing involves the selection of one or more alternatives.

Communicating. Communicating involves the interchange of information from one system to another.

Exchanging. Exchanging involves the interchange of energy and matter between person and environment. Exchanging also involves the transformation of energy from one form to another.

Feeling. Feeling involves a sensing of physical and intuitive awareness.

Knowing. Knowing is the process of personal recognition of self and world.

Moving. Moving is the process of rhythmic alternating between activity and rest.

Perceiving. Perceiving is the process of receiving and interpreting information.

Relating. Relating is the process of connecting with other persons and with the environment.

Valuing. Valuing is the process of assigning worth. (Newman, 1986, p. 74).

Nursing
Nursing is the act of assisting people to utilize the power that is within them as they evolve toward higher levels of consciousness. Nursing is directed toward recognizing the pattern of the person in interaction with the environment and accepting the interaction

as a process of evolving consciousness. Nursing facilitates the process of pattern recognition by a rhythmic connecting of the nurse with the client in an authentic way for the purpose of illuminating the pattern and discovering the new rules of a higher level of organization. Nursing is relating in mutual partnership with a client in the expansion of consciousness (Newman, 1979, p. 67; 1986, p. 68, p. 88; 1990a, p. 40; 1990b, p. 136).

Pattern

Pattern is relatedness. Pattern is characterized by movement, diversity, and rhythm. Pattern is a scheme, a design, or framework, a series of acts and aspects regarded as characteristic of persons or environments. Pattern is seen in person-environment interaction. Pattern is recognized on the basis of variation and may not be seen all at once. Pattern unfolds over time with one configuration evolving into the next configuration and so forth. Pattern is key to understanding reality and is manifest in the way one moves, speaks, talks, and relates with others. Pattern identifies the wholeness of the person (Newman 1986a, p. 14; 1990a, p. 40; 1990b, p. 132).

Pattern Recognition

Pattern recognition is the insight or instantaneous recognition of a principle, a realization of a truth, or reconciliation of a duality. Pattern recognition illuminates the possibilities for action. Pattern recognition is key to the process of evolving to higher levels of consciousness (Newman, 1983a, p. x-xi; 1990a, p. 40).

Person

A person is a dynamic pattern of energy and an open system in interaction with the environment. Persons are identified by their patterns of consciousness. The person does not *possess* consciousness. The person *is* consciousness (Newman, 1986a, p. 33; 1990a, p. 40).

Praxis Research

Praxis research is a process whereby theory, practice, and research are one. Praxis research requires a mutual relationship between interviewee and researcher within a process of inquiry requiring negotiation, reciprocity, and empowerment. In praxis research, the interviewees gain insight into their pattern and concomitant illumination of their action possibilities. An intersection occurs between the interviewee's self-understanding and the researcher's

theoretical stance, which provides a change-enhancing context
(Lather, 1986, p. 262; Newman, 1990a, p. 38).

Space

Space is inextricably linked with time. There is personal space,
inner space, territorial space, shared space, physical and geographical space, maneuverable space, distance-regulating space and life
space (Newman, 1979, p. 61).

Time

Time is inextricably linked with space. There is subjective time,
objective time, time perspective, utilization of time, private time,
coordinated time, and shared time (Newman, 1979, p. 61).

References

Batey, M. (1991). Response: Research as practice. *Nursing Science Quarterly*, *4*(3), 101-103.

Bentov, I. (1978). *Stalking the wild pendulum*. New York: Dutton.

Bohm, D. (1980). *Wholeness and the implicate order*. London: Routledge.

Boyd, C. O. (1990). Critical appraisal of developing nursing research methods. *Nursing Science Quarterly*, *3*(1), 42-43.

Cowling, W. R. (1988). Book reviews: Newman, M. A. (1986). Health as expanding consciousness. *Nursing Science Quarterly*, *1*(3), 133-134.

Fawcett, J. (1989). *Conceptual models of nursing* (2nd ed.). Philadelphia: F. A. Davis.

Flew, A. (Ed.). (1984). *A dictionary of philosophy* (2nd ed.). New York: St. Martin's.

Kalb, K. A. (1990). The gift: Applying Newman's theory of health in nursing practice. In M. E. Parker (Ed.), *Nursing theories in practice* (pp. 163-186). New York: National League for Nursing.

Kim, M. J., & Moritz, D. A. (Eds.). (1982). *Classification of nursing diagnosis: Proceedings of the third and fourth national conferences*. New York: McGraw-Hill.

Klein, S. (1989). Caregiver burden and moral development. *Image*, *21*(2), 94-97.

Kuhn, T. (1970). *The structure of scientific revolutions*. (2nd ed.). Chicago: The University of Chicago Press.

Lather, P. (1986). Research as praxis. *Harvard Educational Review*, *56*(3), 257-277.

Marchione, J. M. (1986a). Application of the new paradigm of health to individuals, families and communities. Special Supplement. In M. Newman (Ed.), *Health as expanding consciousness* (pp. 107-134). St. Louis: C. V. Mosby.

Marchione, J. M. (1986b). Pattern as methodology for assessing family health: Newman's theory of health. In P. Winstead-Fry (Ed.), *Case studies in nursing theory* (pp. 215-240). New York: National League for Nursing.

Moch, S. D. (1990). Health within the experience of breast cancer. *Journal of Advanced Nursing*, *15*, 1426-1435.

44

Moss, R. (1981). *The I that is we*. Millbrae, CA: Celestial Arts.

Newman, M. A. (1966). Identifying patient needs in short-span nurse-patient relationships. *Nursing Forum, 5*(1), 76-86.

Newman, M. A. (1972). Time estimation in relation to gait tempo. *Perceptual and Motor Skills, 34*, 359-366.

Newman, M. A. (1976). Movement tempo and the experience of time. *Nursing Research, 25*, 273-279.

Newman, M. A. (1979). *Theory development in nursing*. Philadelphia: F. A. Davis.

Newman, M. A. (1982). Time as an index of consciousness with age. *Nursing Research 31*, 290-293.

Newman, M. A. (1983a). Editorial. *Advances in Nursing Science, 5*(2), x-xi.

Newman, M. A. (1983b). Newman's health theory. In I. Clements & F. Roberts (Eds.), *Family health: A theoretical approach to nursing care* (pp. 161-175). New York: Wiley.

Newman, M. A. (1983c). The continuing revolution: A history of nursing science. In N. L. Chaska (Ed.), *The nursing profession: A time to speak* (pp. 385-393). New York: McGraw-Hill.

Newman, M. A. (1984). Nursing diagnosis: Looking at the whole. *American Journal of Nursing, 84*, 1496-1499.

Newman, M. A. (1986). *Health as expanding consciousness*. St. Louis: Mosby.

Newman, M. A. (1987). Patterning. In M. Duffy & N. J. Pender (Eds.), *Conceptual issues in health promotion: Report of proceedings of a wingspread conference* (pp. 36-50). Indianapolis: Sigma Theta Tau.

Newman, M. A. (1990a). Newman's theory of health as praxis. *Nursing Science Quarterly, 3*(1), 37-41.

Newman, M. A. (1990b). Shifting to higher consciousness. In M. Parker (Ed.), *Nursing theories in practice* (pp. 129-139). New York: National League for Nursing.

Newman, M. A. (1991). Commentary: Research as practice. *Nursing Science Quarterly, 4*(3), 100.

Newman, M. A., & Gaudiano, J. K. (1984). Depression as an explanation for decreased subjective time in the elderly. *Nursing Research, 33*(3), 137-139.

Newman, M. A., Lamb, G. S., & Michaels, C. (1991). Nurse case management: The coming together of theory and practice. *Nursing and Health Care, 12*(8), 404-408.

Newman, M. A., & Moch, S. D. (in press). Life patterns of persons with coronary heart disease. *Nursing Science Quarterly*.

Pearson, B. D. (1988). Book reviews: Newman, M. A. (1986). Health as expanding consciousness. *Nursing Science Quarterly, 1*(3), 134-136.

Ray, M. A. (1990). Critical reflective analysis of Parse's and Newman's research methodologies. *Nursing Science Quarterly, 3*(1), 44-46.

Robinson, K. M. (1990). Predictors of burden among wife caregivers. *Scholarly Inquiry for Nursing Practice: An International Journal, 4*(3), 189-203.

Rogers, M. E. (1970). *An introduction to the theoretical basis of nursing*. Philadelphia: F. A. Davis.

Schorr, J. A., Farnham, R. C., & Ervin, S. M. (1991). Health patterns in aging women as expanding consciousness. *Advances in Nursing Science, 13*(4), 52-63.

Silva, M. C. (1988). Book Reviews: Newman, M. A. (1986). Health as Expanding Consciousness. *Nursing Science Quarterly, 1*(3), 136-138.

Smith, M. C. (1990). Pattern in nursing practice. *Nursing Science Quarterly, 3*(2), 57-59.

Teilhard de Chardin, P. (1959). *The phenomenon of man.* New York: Harper & Brothers.

Watson, J. (1987). Book reviews: Health as expanding consciousness. *Journal of Professional Nursing, 3*(5), 387.

West, M. C. (1984). *Patterns of health in mothers of developmentally disabled children.* Unpublished master's thesis. The Pennsylvania State University, University Park, PA.

Young, A. (1976a). *The geometry of meaning.* San Francisco: Robert Briggs.

Young, A. M. (1976b). *The reflexive universe: Evolution of consciousness.* San Francisco: Robert Briggs.

Bibliography

Theory Development—Classic and Contemporary Works

Newman, M. A. (1979). *Theory development in nursing*. Philadelphia: F. A. Davis.
Newman, M. A. (1983a). Editorial. *Advances in Nursing Science*, 5(2), x-xi.
Newman, M. A. (1983b). Newman's health theory. In I. Clements & F. Roberts (Eds.), *Family health: A theoretical approach to nursing care* (pp. 161-175). New York: Wiley.
Newman, M. A. (1984). Nursing diagnosis: Looking at the whole. *American Journal of Nursing*, 84, 1496-1499.
Newman, M. A. (1986). *Health as expanding consciousness*. St. Louis: Mosby.
Newman, M. A. (1987a). Nursing's emerging paradigm: The diagnosis of pattern. In A. M. McLane (Ed.), *Classification of nursing diagnoses: Proceedings of the seventh conference*, North American Nursing Diagnosis Association (pp. 53-60). St. Louis: Mosby.
Newman, M. A. (1987b). Patterning. In M. Duffy & N. J. Pender (Eds.), *Conceptual issues in health promotion: Report of proceedings of a wingspread conference* (pp.36-50). Indianapolis: Sigma Theta Tau.
Newman, M. A. (1989). The spirit of nursing. *Holistic Nursing Practice*, 3(3), 1-6.
Newman, M. A. (1990a). Newman's theory of health as praxis. *Nursing Science Quarterly*, 3(1), 37-41.
Newman, M. A. (1990b). Shifting to higher consciousness. In M. E. Parker (Ed.), *Nursing theories in practice* (pp. 129-139). New York: National League for Nursing.
Newman, M. A. (1990c). Professionalism: Myth or reality. In N. L. Chaska (Ed.), *The nursing profession: Turning points* (pp. 49-52). St. Louis: Mosby.
Newman, M. A. (1991). Commentary: Research as practice. *Nursing Science Quarterly*, 4(3), 100.
Newman, M. A. (1979). Movement, time, and the experience of health. *Research*, 15, 273-279.

Newman, M. A., Lamb, G. S., & Michaels, C. (1991). Nurse case management: The coming together of theory and practice. *Nursing and Health Care, 12*(8), 404-408.
Newman, M. A., & Moch, S. D. (in press). Life patterns of persons with coronary heart disease. *Nursing Science Quarterly.*

Influencing Sources

Bentov, I. (1978). *Stalking the wild pendulum.* New York: Dutton.
Bohm, D. (1980). *Wholeness and the implicate order.* London: Routledge.
Lather, P. (1986). Research as praxis. *Harvard Educational Review, 56*(3), 257-277.
Moss, R. (1981). *The I that is we.* Millbrae, CA.: Celestial Arts.
Rogers, M. E. (1970). *An introduction to the theoretical basis of nursing.* Philadelphia: F.A. Davis.
Teilhard de Chardin, P. (1959). *The phenomenon of man.* New York: Harper & Brothers.
Young, A. M. (1976a). *The geometry of meaning.* San Francisco: Robert Briggs.
Young, A. M. (1976b). *The reflexive universe: Evolution of consciousness.* San Francisco: Robert Briggs.

Research and Application References

Gustafson, W. (1990). Application of Newman's theory of health: Pattern recognition as nursing practice. In M. E. Parker (Ed.), *Nursing theories in practice* (pp. 141-161). New York: National League for Nursing.
Kalb, K. A. (1990). The gift: Applying Newman's theory of health in nursing practice. In M. E. Parker (Ed.), *Nursing theories in practice* (pp. 163-186). New York: National League for Nursing.
Jonsdottir, H. (1988). *Health patterns of clients with chronic obstructive pulmonary disease,* Unpublished master's thesis. University of Minnesota, Minneapolis.
Marchione, J. M. (1986a). Application of the new paradigm of health to individuals, families and communities. Special Supplement in M. Newman, *Health as expanding consciousness* (pp. 107-134). St. Louis: Mosby.
Marchione, J. M. (1986b). Pattern as methodology for assessing family health: Newman's theory of health. In P. Winstead-Fry, (Ed.), *Case studies in nursing theory* (pp. 215-240). New York: National League for Nursing.
Moch, S. D. (1988). *Health in illness: Experiences with breast cancer* (Doctoral dissertation, University of Minnesota). Dissertation Abstracts International *50,* 47 b.
Moch, S. D. (1990). Health within the experience of breast cancer. *Journal of Advanced Nursing, 15,* 1426-1435.
Newman, M. A. (1966). Identifying patient needs in short span nurse-patient relationships. *Nursing Forum, 5*(1), 76-86.
Newman, M. A. (1972). Time estimation in relation to gait tempo. *Perceptual and Motor Skills, 34,* 359-366.
Newman, M. A. (1976). Movement tempo and the experience of time. *Nursing Research, 25,* 273-279.

Newman, M. A. (1982). Time as an index of consciousness with age. *Nursing Research, 31*, 290-293.

Newman, M. A. (1991). Commentary: Research as practice. *Nursing Science Quarterly, 4*(3), 100.

Newman, M. A., & Gaudiano, J. K. (1984). Depression as an explanation for decreased subjective time in the elderly. *Nursing Research, 33*(3), 137-139.

Newman, M. A., Lamb, G. L., & Michaels, C. (1991). Nurse case management: The coming together of theory and practice. *Nursing and Health Care, 12* (8), 404-408.

Newman, M. A., & Moch, S. D. (in press). Life patterns of persons with coronary heart disease. (Accepted for publication in *Nursing Science Quarterly*).

Schorr, J. A., Farnham, R. C., & Ervin, S. M. (1991). Health patterns in aging women as expanding consciousness. *Advances in Nursing Science, 13*(4), 52-63.

West, M. C. (1984). *Patterns of health in mothers of developmentally disabled children.* Unpublished master's thesis. The Pennsylvania State University, University Park, PA.

Critique of Newman's Theory

Batey, M. (1991). Response: Research as practice. *Nursing Science Quarterly, 4*(3), 101-103.

Boyd, C. O. (1990). Critical appraisal of developing nursing research methods. *Nursing Science Quarterly, 3*(1), 42-43.

Cowling, W. R. (1988). Book reviews: Newman, M. A. (1986). Health as expanding consciousness. *Nursing Science Quarterly, 1*(3), 133-134.

Pearson, B. D. (1988). Book reviews: Newman, M. A. (1986). Health as expanding consciousness. *Nursing Science Quarterly, 1*(3), 134-136.

Ray, M. A. (1990). Critical reflective analysis of Parse's and Newman's research methodologies. *Nursing Science Quarterly, 3*(1), 44-46.

Silva, M. C. (1988). Book reviews: Newman, M. A. (1986). Health as expanding consciousness. *Nursing Science Quarterly, 1*(3), 136-138.

Smith, M. C. (1990). Pattern in nursing practice. *Nursing Science Quarterly, 3*(2), 57-59.

Watson, J. (1987). Book reviews: Health as expanding consciousness. *Journal of Professional Nursing, 3*(5), 387.

Videotapes

Helene Fuld Health Trust (Producer), & Fawcett, J. (Interviewer). (1990). *Portraits of excellence: Margaret Newman.* [VHS videocassette]. Oakland, CA: Studio III.

Kerr, J. (Director). (1990). *Interview of Margaret Newman.* Part of a series of Nursing as a Practical Science, Edmonton, Alberta, Canada. Available from the University of Alberta, Faculty of Nursing.

Stearns, S. (Producer), & Marchione, J. (Interviewer). (1983). *A conversation with Margaret Newman, explaining her theory of health.* JVC videocassette. Available

from the University of Minnesota, School of Nursing; The Pennsylvania
State University, Division of Nursing; and the University of Akron, College of Nursing.

About the Author

◆

Joanne Marchione is a scholar of theories related to health and human caring. For more than a decade she has explored theory development and application with students from nursing and other disciplines. She has also mentored and advised faculty on the application of theory and praxis research.

Professor Marchione received a baccalaureate degree from Frances Payne Bolton School of Nursing, Case Western Reserve University. Her graduate degrees are in education and anthropology with an emphasis on nursing science. Over the years she has focused on a multicultural approach to the health of families and children. She has studied at many universities in the United States, Europe, and Canada in a continued effort to improve her teaching relative to higher education, theories, cultural diversity, health, child and family health, and nursing. She received certification from the University of Washington to teach parent-child interpersonal and environmental assessment skills.

She has studied child health, family health, and comparative health systems. She has presented her findings to local, national, and international professional assemblies. Currently, she is studying children in homeless family situations.